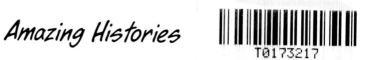

Amazing Histories

THE AMAZING HISTORY OF
MEDICINE

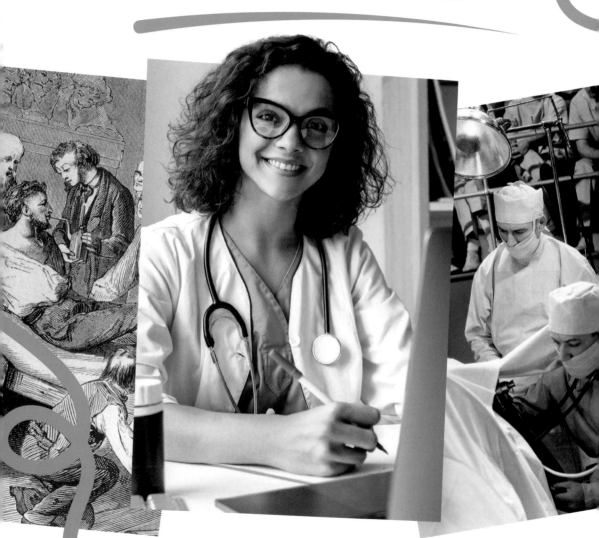

BY HEATHER MURPHY CAPPS

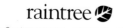

raintree 🦫

a Capstone company — publishers for children

Raintree is an imprint of Capstone Global Library Limited, a company incorporated in England and Wales having its registered office at 264 Banbury Road, Oxford, OX2 7DY – Registered company number: 6695582

www.raintree.co.uk
myorders@raintree.co.uk

Edited by Alison Deering
Designed by: Jaime Willems
Media research by: Donna Metcalf;
Production by: Tori Abraham
Originated by Capstone Global Library Ltd
Printed and bound in India

ISBN 978 1 3982 5149 6 (hardback)
ISBN 978 1 3982 5150 2 (paperback)

British Library Cataloguing in Publication Data
A full catalogue record for this book is available from the British Library.

Acknowledgements
We would like to thank the following for permission to reproduce photographs: Alamy: Hamza Khan, 19, Pictorial Press Ltd, 23 top, Science History Images, 8, 11, 15, 17, 18, 21; Getty Images: ilbusca, 24-25; Shutterstock: apichart sripa, 6, Daniel Chetroni, 29, Emilio100, 7, Everett Collection, cover, 1, left and right, back cover top left, New Africa, 9, Peakstock, 13, 27, peterfactors, cover top left, 30, Prostock-studio, back cover middle left, 5, Shutter_M, 10, Stock 4you, cover, 1 middle, Wikimedia: National Library of Medicine, 23 bottom

Every effort has been made to contact copyright holders of material reproduced in this book. Any omissions will be rectified in subsequent printings if notice is given to the publisher.

All the internet addresses (URLs) given in this book were valid at the time of going to press. However, due to the dynamic nature of the internet, some addresses may have changed, or sites may have changed or ceased to exist since publication. While the author and publisher regret any inconvenience this may cause readers, no responsibility for any such changes can be accepted by either the author or the publisher.

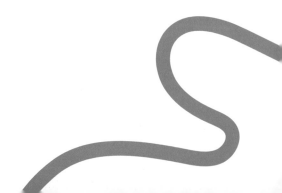

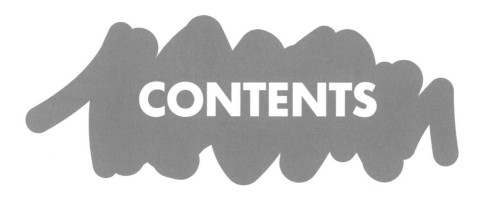

CONTENTS

Words in **BOLD** are in the glossary.

THE DOCTOR WILL
SEE YOU NOW

No one likes to be ill. It was even worse to be ill in ancient times. People tried some very strange cures. Let's look at the amazing history of medicine.

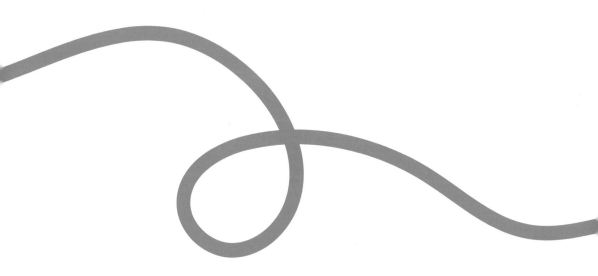

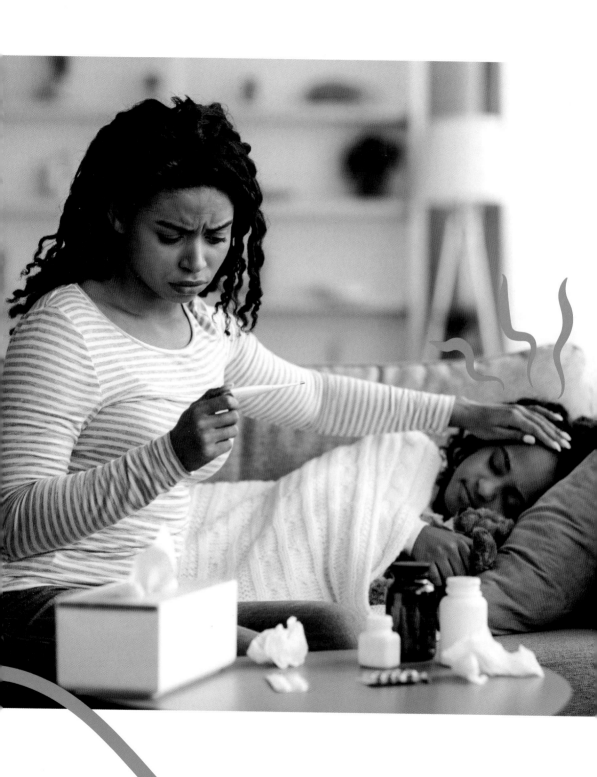

EARLY
MEDICINE

Nobody is sure when medicine first began.
Ancient people didn't keep written records.
They also didn't go to medical school. They
often thought angry gods made people ill.

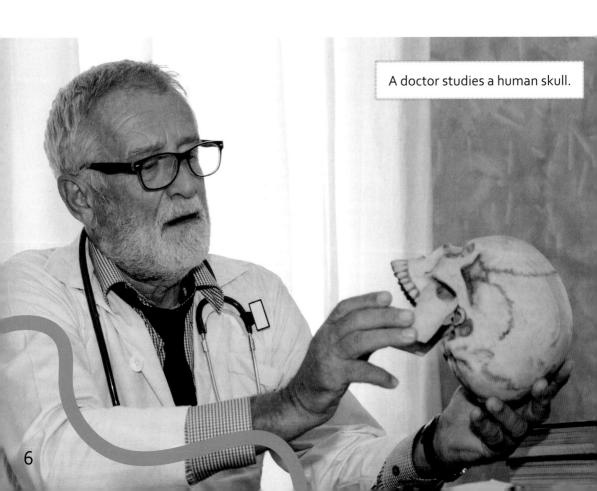

A doctor studies a human skull.

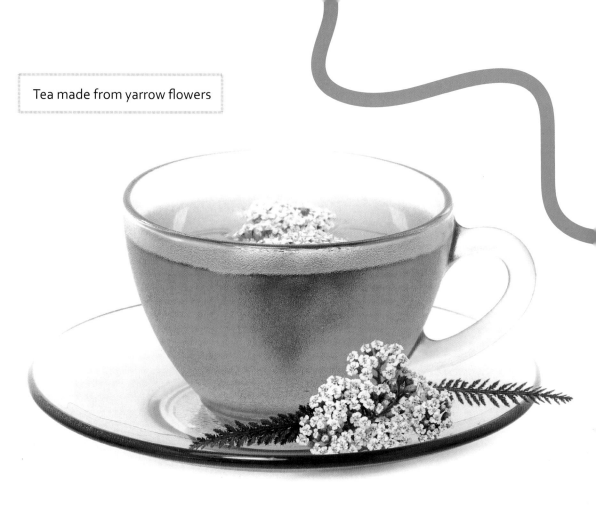

Tea made from yarrow flowers

Healers used natural cures. People chewed
plants, such as yarrow, to help with stomach ache.

Ayurveda

Doctors created **Ayurveda** more than 3,000 years ago. The word means "knowledge of life". This natural system of health started in India. It is still used today.

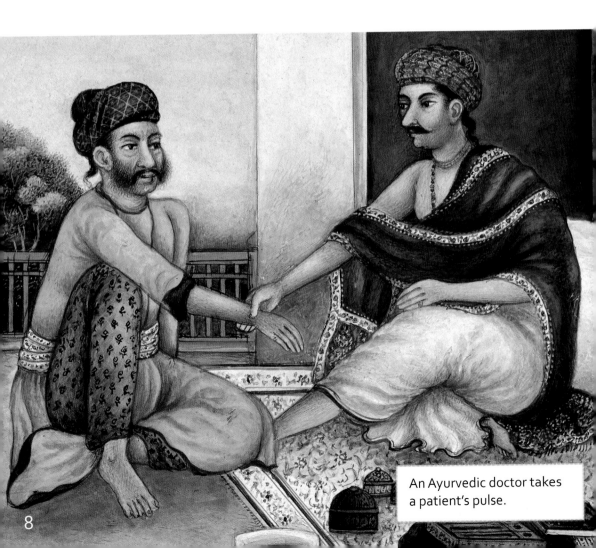

An Ayurvedic doctor takes a patient's pulse.

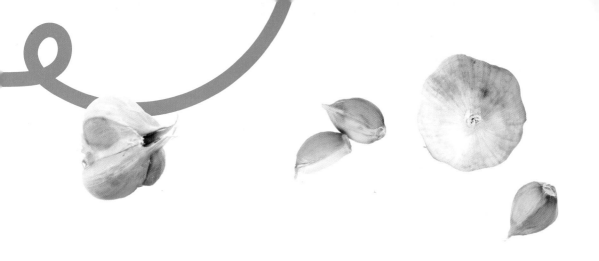

Doctors encourage good health. They tell people to exercise and eat a balanced diet. To stay healthy, people also use foods such as garlic and ginger.

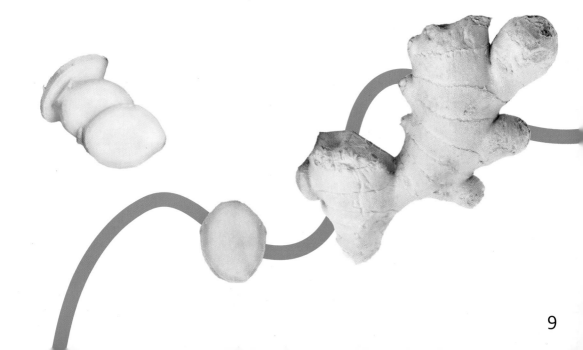

ANCIENT
ADVANCES

Doctors in ancient Egypt made a special tea. They made it from willow tree bark and leaves. The tea helped headaches, sore muscles and fevers. Honey was used on wounds. It killed germs.

Egyptian doctors wrote down their methods. These are some of the first ever medical records.

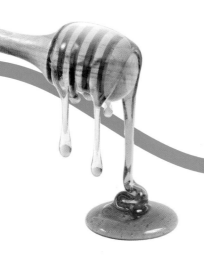

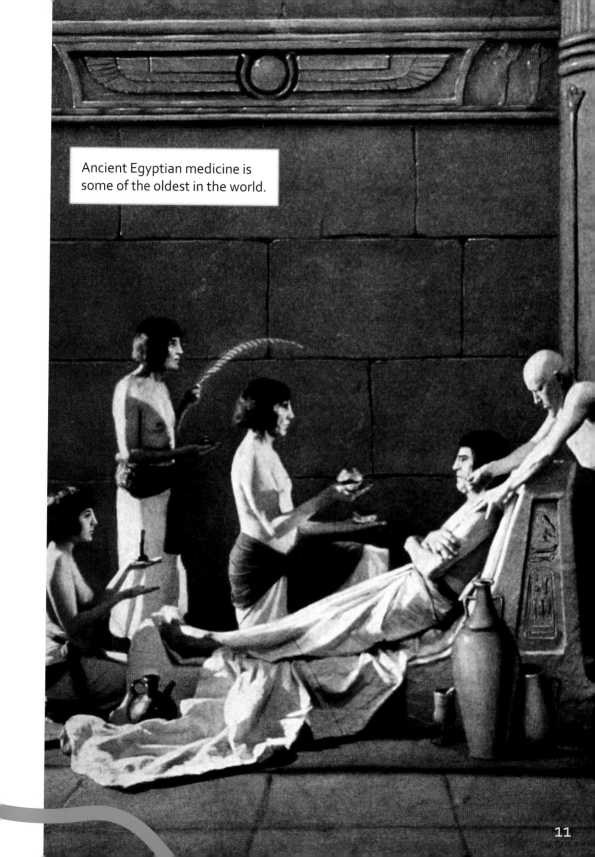

Ancient Egyptian medicine is some of the oldest in the world.

Acupuncture

In ancient China, doctors used **acupuncture**. They stuck tiny needles in different parts of the body. They even put needles in people's faces or ears. Ouch!

The needles seem to help. Some doctors still use them today. They say this method unblocks stuck energy. It helps fix headaches, sore muscles and some illnesses.

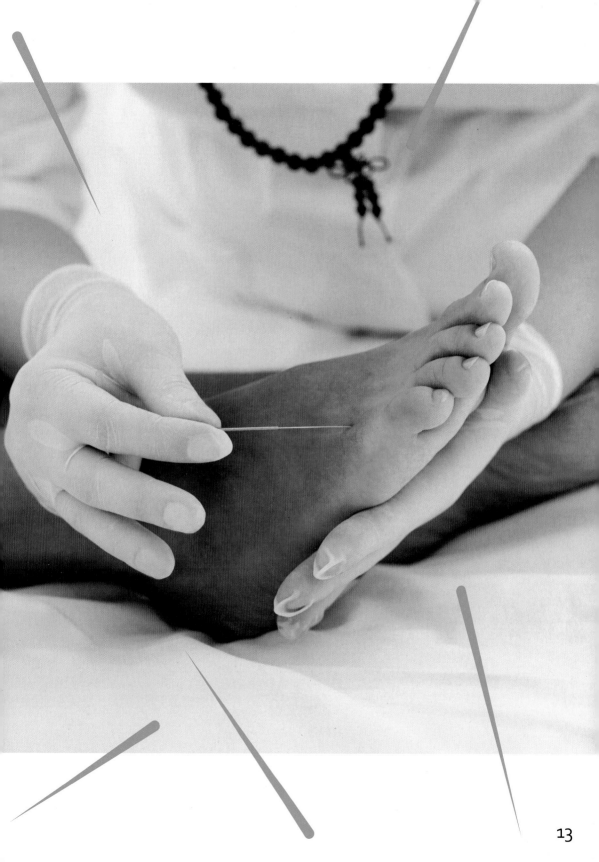

FINDING
BALANCE

Ancient Greek medicine was called **humorism**. But doctors weren't laughing. They believed people had fluids in their bodies called humours. These included blood, yellow **bile**, black bile and **phlegm**.

The Greeks believed that these fluids had to be balanced. They tried to help people in some revolting ways. They made people throw up or have diarrhoea. Yuck!

DID YOU KNOW?

Hippocrates is known as the father of modern medicine. The Hippocratic oath, versions of which many medical schools still use, is named after him.

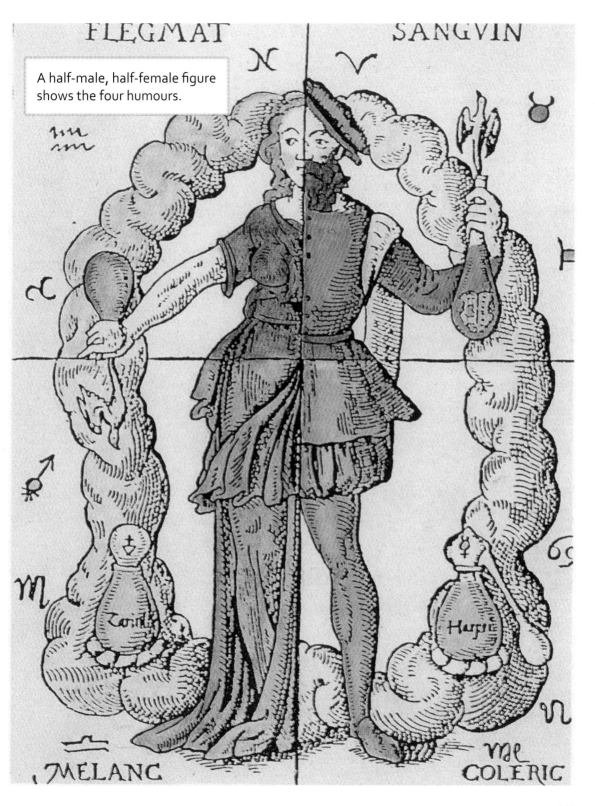

FLEGMAT

SANGVIN

A half-male, half-female figure shows the four humours.

MELANC

COLERIC

Bloodletting

Some ancient doctors also used bloodletting. They made cuts in a person's veins to drain blood. They thought that this helped with balancing the humours.

This process was dangerous. In 1685, King Charles II had a stroke. Doctors drained about 550 ml (1 pint) of his blood. The king died.

DID YOU KNOW?

George Washington, the first president of the United States, also died after bloodletting. Doctors drained nearly 40 per cent of his blood.

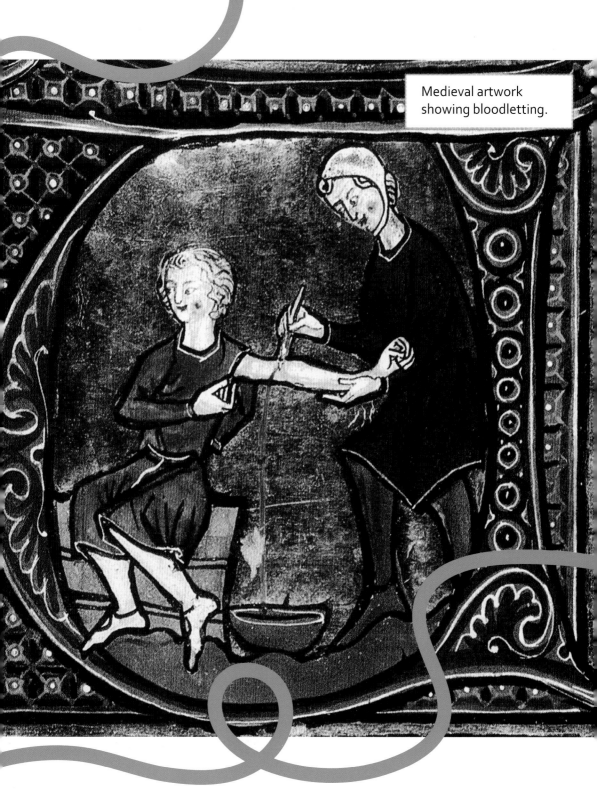

Medieval artwork showing bloodletting.

OLD-SCHOOL
OPERATIONS

One of the oldest known operations is a type of brain surgery. It was first done nearly 8,000 years ago. Doctors drilled a small hole into a person's skull. Yikes! They thought this could fix bad headaches, mental illness and more.

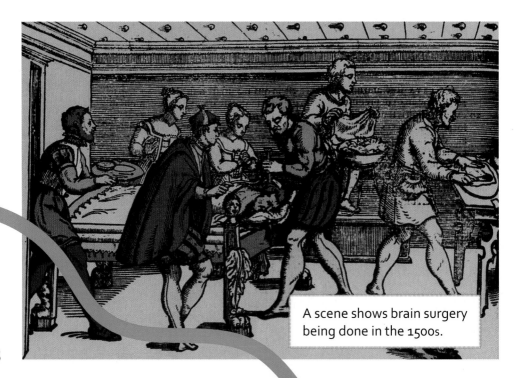

A scene shows brain surgery being done in the 1500s.

A human skull shows evidence of brain surgery.

Plastic surgery

Plastic surgery isn't new. The first nose job was done in India in 600 **BCE**.

Back then, criminals sometimes had their noses cut off. An Indian doctor learned how to help these people. He used skin from a cheek to make a new nose.

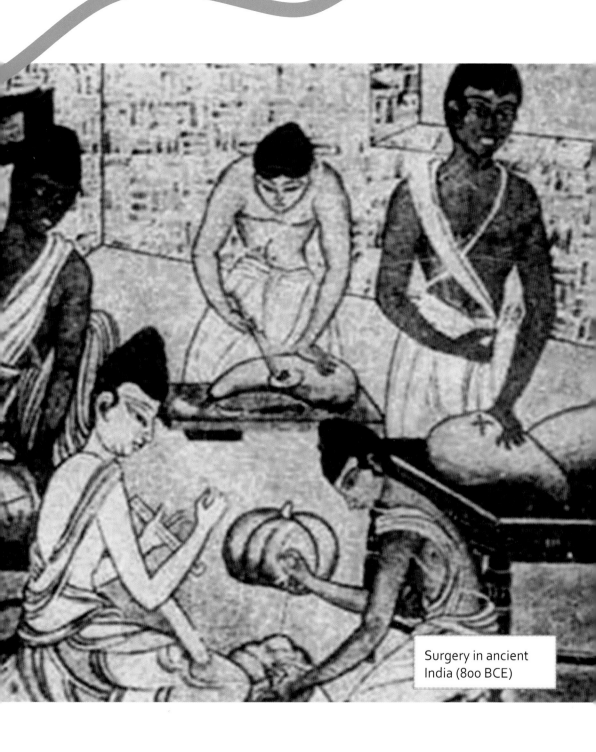

Surgery in ancient India (800 BCE)

MEDICAL
FIRSTS

Italy's School of Salerno was the first medical school. It taught doctors from all over Europe. It was the first school to allow women to study and teach medicine.

Trotula was a doctor and teacher at the school. She wrote an important book on women's health. Some of her teachings are still used today.

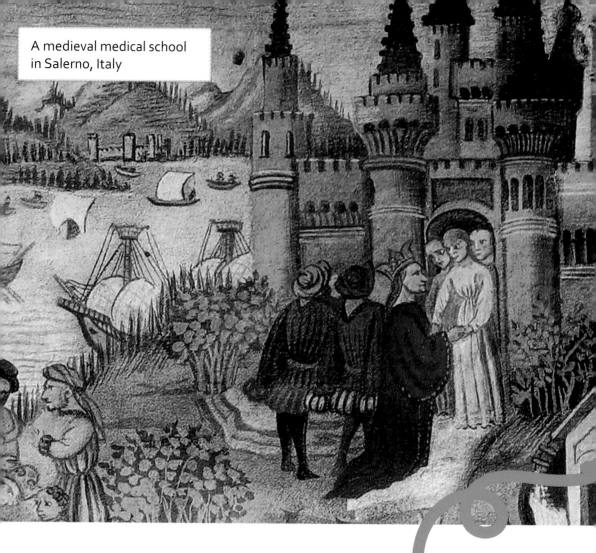

A medieval medical school in Salerno, Italy

DID YOU KNOW?

Elizabeth Blackwell was the first woman to attend medical school in the United States. She graduated from New York's Geneva Medical College in 1850.

In the UK, Elizabeth Garrett Anderson was the first woman to qualify as a doctor in 1865.

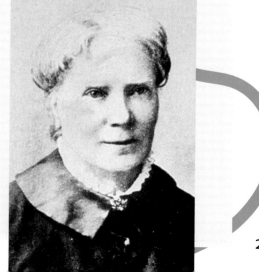

Elizabeth Blackwell

Human dissection

Doctors didn't always know a lot about the human body. They first studied the bodies of animals to learn. But that led to *a lot* of wrong information. In the 1300s, studying dead human bodies was allowed.

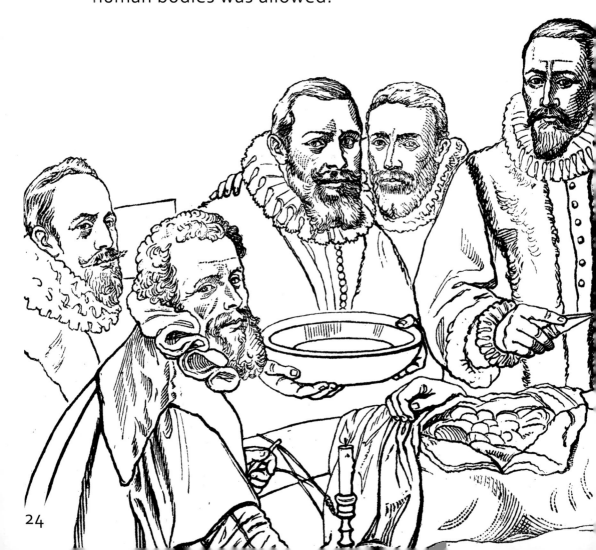

Most people didn't want doctors to cut up dead relatives. Grave robbers dug up bodies instead. They sold the dead to medical schools.

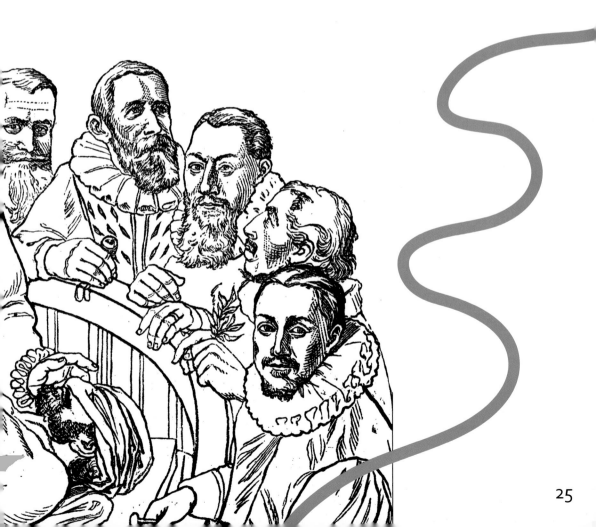

Laughing gas

Controlling pain during surgery wasn't always possible. But in the mid-1800s, doctors tried something new. They used **nitrous oxide**. This is also called laughing gas. People felt no pain after breathing this. Doctors could perform more operations.

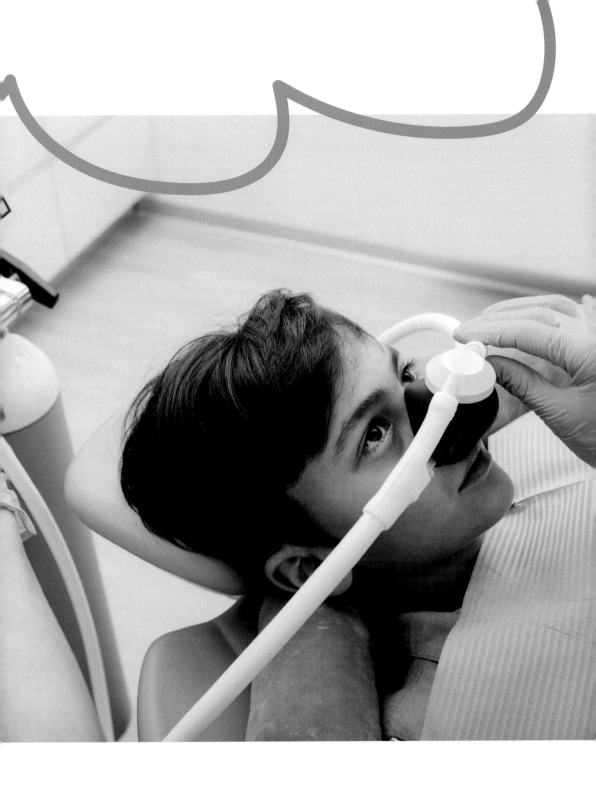

PANDEMICS
AND
VACCINES

In 430 BCE, a **plague** hit Athens, Greece. It was history's first **pandemic**. The disease was caused by bacteria spread by fleas and lice.

DID YOU KNOW?

During the Great Plague of London in 1665, doctors told people to breathe in smelly farts for protection. They believed it could keep people from getting ill!

Antibiotic medicines were created in the 1930s. They treated infections. Today, **vaccines** protect us against many diseases. These include measles, smallpox and more. Hooray for modern medicine!

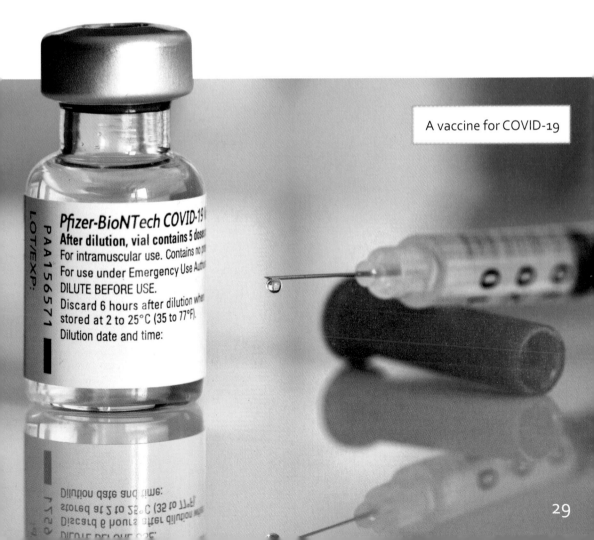

A vaccine for COVID-19

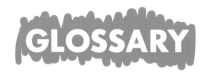

GLOSSARY

acupuncture stimulation of certain points in the body by piercing the skin with metal needles

antibiotic drug that kills bacteria and is used to cure infections and disease

Ayurveda ancient Indian system of medicine

BCE dates before the birth of Christ; these count backwards, so 3000 BCE is earlier than 2500 BCE

bile green liquid that is made by the liver and helps digest food

humorism outdated Greek theory of medicine that is based on balancing four bodily fluids

nitrous oxide gas made up of nitrogen and oxygen; it is used to kill pain during surgery and is also called "laughing gas"

pandemic disease that spreads over a wide area and affects many people

phlegm thick mucus that is produced when someone has a cold

plague disease that spreads quickly and kills most people who catch it

vaccine medicine that prevents a disease

FIND OUT MORE

BOOKS

A Short, Illustrated History of Medicine, John C Miles (Franklin Watts, 2021)

Do No Harm: A Painful History of Medicine, Nick Arnold (Welbeck, 2021)

Medicine: A Magnificently Illustrated History, Briony Hudson (Big Picture, 2022)

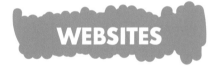

WEBSITES

www.bbc.co.uk/bitesize/topics/zwqqm39/articles/zjrhn9q
Learn about early pandemics on the BBC Bitesize website.

www.youtube.com/watch?v=ogUNkyk3qgI
Find out about historical healthcare with the Horrible Histories team.

INDEX

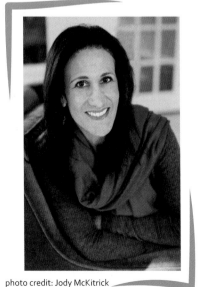

photo credit: Jody McKitrick

ABOUT THE AUTHOR

Heather Murphy Capps is from Minnesota, USA. She spent 20 years as a television news journalist before deciding to focus on her favourite kind of writing: books for children, involving history, social justice, science, magic and a touch of mystery. She's a mixed-race author committed to diversity in publishing, an administrator/contributor to the blog From the Mixed-Up Files . . . of Middle-Grade Authors and the author of the children's novel *Indigo and Ida*. Heather now lives in northern Virginia with her husband, two children and two cats.